Broken Glass in Wet Sand

Hard and Soft Poems

By Ray Scott

Library of Congress Control Number 2011900096

Dewey Decimal 811.54 Scot

Publisher   Clean Table Books
                     1905 Alexandria PK
                     Highland Heights, KY 41076

Email: CTBooksAndCDs@gmail.com:
www.CTBooksAndCDs.com

Cover Design Ray Scott

Thank You

Sue Bayes, Kimberly Sloan, Maribeth Hibbett, Marsha Meadows, John Weyer, Kyle Meadows, Debbie Schaeffer

Who helped with the most difficult part of the writing the reading and critique. The readers helped in many stages of writing and development. Without them this work would have been lacking.

Thank You
Campbell County, Ky. Library Staff and Resources those were essential to the production of this book.

Dedicated to the readers without
whom there would be no book

Introduction

An introduction to a book of poems is not really necessary the poems survive as their own introduction. Logically as each poem stands alone maybe they all need an introduction. Maybe one introduction for each poem?

Most poets write because they are compelled to write. A name for the process could be to Poet. Or Poets Poet. There are many poets out there poeting Hundreds of chapbook printers/publishers. The real reward is that the audience is the beginning and crown of poetry expressions. Poets are valid in the terms of "who will read it" and "how does it feel" the payoff is that the words are clear and valued by the reader. Poets are sometimes in the processes of beginning to change the language or making events/people real as life.

This book is for those who want to appreciate the trials of the mentally challenged individuals. The writer is Bipolar and has enjoyed over thirty years of successful functioning. As you likely know Bipolar is a lifelong struggle. In addition to being bipolar the author has been a Social Worker, Counselor, and Mental Health Technician. The soft poems that are happy and playful are largely the result of effective/affective treatment and Bipolar Medication

Some of the hard poems are the result of personal experience in coping with severe depression, mania, insomnia, and suicide. The hard poems on Schizophrenia, Child Abuse, Incest, and Drug Addiction are the result of years of clinical, counseling and Social Profession experience with victims of the same.   The patients/clients/places are thoroughly fictionalized. The events and affects and mental orientations are very real.

The soft poems are written as the celebration of sanity. Many beautiful things happen when someone leaves most of the "madness" behind.

Contents

All Hail ee Cummings

Sleepless

normal time does not count
when there is nothing else to do

free tears spell exhaustion
tired
so hours pass with a low score

wires stretch from my head
each wire touches a part of brain
and dangles out into the ceiling and room
invisible light is at each end of the wire

minutes go by without names
the clock keeps the score

there is a blue wind just before dawn
that only those who watch the whole night are able to see

a dog barks alone

Sleep is a just in case death
you get to die but not for good

To not sleep is to become insane with most wits at end
split seconds merge
a second passes an hour creeps by
too numb to count

is it 3am or noon???

sometimes the light stings

Sleepless 2

quiet cats stalk creatures sheltered by the night

there is a clicking noise that means a roach is pacing
roaches scatter in just visible sounds
dark lumps across the floor
big enough in the half light
to look like mice running

the Brain is an open box
allowing undigested thoughts to enter

the Brain talks back and forth
remember forget remember
night time is the best time to remember quiet fights
even those with every day friends

sleep whispers
again again again
nothing else matters
sleep to stay alive

stay awake is written in specks of crumbled stone

you can learn to hear flies wings
mostly in hot months
when there is nothing else to do

Quiet sounds seem like drums
hours pass with a low score
too numb to count too numb to count too numb to count

Death is no stranger
Just a choice

All the Saints

All the prayers to all the Saints
did not make one guilty priest
keep his pants on
victim youngsters new to Jesus
wearing miniature hassocks

the quiet solemn moments
hazy with Latin and Greek
did not compel the sitting bishops
to protect the children

Instead
the abusers were sent
to different tall houses
to find new and better targets
new and better boys and girls
Some innocent priests looked away
and did no deeds to save a child

There shall be a place on the mill stone
for those who failed to see (who knew nothing)
when it is cast into the sea

Some racked with guilt
ended their life
that did nothing
for the unsheltered victim children

All the prayers to all the Saints did nothing
to make a guilty priest
keep his pants on

Meeting

meeting you
when the sky is bright red
and the flowers of summer
touch a happy nose

gently we touch the grass
and listen to the warm breezes
holding us next to soul
looking at innocence

needing you
is a small prayer

holding you under the evening star
silence of the noisy night
eyes that see in the dark

slow paced steps
under a half hidden moon

rocks form a castle
leaves shine in the moonlight
quiet love in wind breeze bushes
silent words in hand touch

breath as close as my own
warmth from gentle nearness
and tomorrow is yet to be

Color the Wall

pick it up stupid
spilled two gallons of vegetable soup

now you'll be on a talking ban
respect your team leader
don't talk about him
and the grade school kids

Sedra wants to kill you
and it's your entire fault
you keep remembering you used to be a counselor
you aren't here to listen to problems

your roommate says you talk about getting out
but that's not what the judge says

you told Jean she doesn't belong here
she says she isn't guilty
and you believe that

we want you to know
you've been doing a lot of good work here

you're just a medicine cabinet junky
admit you'd like to do Susan

Stay and get the help you need
Actually the Greyhound bus driver
was more help

The Brain is an open box
allowing undigested thoughts to enter

hazy faces with dark eyes
pictures
in faded colors
wrong colors
right picture

dripping moments
old stories made of triangle shapes
chills
passing by necks

sans friends
sans associates
sans enemies

the box is open
the good song of life
enters

a bird floats by/passes
an elephant sings
a tree turns bright red
misty grass turns wet green
sunlight dances across the field

the brain is open
to warm words
friends and lovers
alive

broken glass in wet sand

some poems are written with the flourish of a fountain pen
and spread words of cheer

history remembers some poets
their poems written by feather with a bottle of ink

some poems rhyme in meter and style
some are pointed with capitols left out
or misspelled

a part of many poems are neatly nearly written
on old crumbled napkins on a bar room table
the wrinkles match the poet's eyes

some poems are too brutal to print
unless dotted out with broken glass bottles
smeared in the wet sand

with...............
               left out souls
               left out names
               left out lies
               rhyming facts

these poems are written with broken glass in wet sand

So I got in my car

The oil company is oiling the ocean
putting oil on top of blue sea water

So I got in my car
and went and saw the reed slick beach

Birds are dying in the black death syrup

So I got in my car
and went to help the rescuers

Ten thousand people can not go out in their boats
to find the sea and fish

So I got in my car
and went to see the protest

The beach where I work is closed

So I got in my car
to go apply for Unemployment benefits
So I got in my car

THE AIR bleeds the smell of oil
It is everywhere nowhere left to go
Nowhere to hide

I drove out to see the blimp
taking pictures of the soaked slimy oily sea
So I got in my car

Singing Voice

A voice like singing
warmth in her eyes

teeth that laugh

just one day became
twenty six years

more beauty than all the shiny statues
more gentle compassion than two other people

fine fingers knitting
new things from old designs
grimy hands from garden parts
tired hands from constant weaving
rested hands from daily reading
power hands from heavy lifting

her smile is electric it is contagious
her modes range in beauty to peaceful
to anger and quickly back

a warm place under the blankets
a soft kiss that says
I love and respect you
and the person that you are

she is the best part of life
sometimes you just get it right

a touch of blonde hair looking red in the sun
blue buttons on a white blouse

warm touches of soft hands
quiet whispers

so many little things to say
so many words
to mean it

leaning on a tree
skipping rocks
across the water

searching for old bottles
in the dark mud
there used to be a brick house
quiet words
the loud happy

happy tears slow smiles

just as we are

a warm bed
busy white legs
holding tight

A moment of peace
and a harmonica and piano concert for two

Mr sir get some sleep

You can't practice karate kicks on hospital ward walls.

Get some sleep.

"Nobody ever died from lack of sleep"

Eyes feel like brown sand
too dry to rub DEEP WORDS
the poet is on leave
but never stops

it's all words and pills.
The pills are scheduled
the words
never stop

Lie awake
truth awake
never stop

If they call you mister
you have to call them doctor or nurse
never stop

the labels are
never stopped
never stopping
never stop

The clock strikes the square at midnight

they pulled john number seventeen
from the brown river water
his body leaking liquid mud and bloody water
probably a bridge jumper

no one gets out of the black plastic bag
TAG NO 563 Jones

inside the beating streets rhythm

a sore black man
rides sleeping on the bus
to where how often unknown

fifty cents
for a few naps away from the heat of day
until the driver notices

at the brown river
no one gets out without the black plastic bag

lucky number tag no 564
a few minutes to like television
until the manager clears the sidewalk window
the number 564
my number is next

Mocking Man

mocking man
with all yellow and jagged teeth
mean teeth

a barely warm tan raincoat almost black
have to do for winter
canvas shoes with newspaper inserts walk on yesterday's news
or next month's investment

wants a meal bad but not from
parish kitchen

too many noodles
not enough salt
no real tomatoes

one day three days ago

found a mostly uneaten big mac
good meal that week

going to mother saint's mission
named for Mary Magalin or something like that
get a bath and clean my clothes

old clean clothes are best for money asking
sign will work for food helps sometimes
sleeping in a warm pipe beneath the white bridge
a cardboard box will stop the cold from the ground

sleep is the only peace

Mocking Man 2

I have a dog sometimes
his name is Street
he shares my food
it's not enough
Street has begging territory
just like me

some time

There's enough change
for a bottle of Mad Dog 20 20
for a little while
the world goes away

I called my son
he lives in Memphis
he still remembers
the pain I caused my family
I can remember nothing better

If you hide well
the police
won't find you at night

it is now too cold to sleep
move hands just to breathe
still holding an
empty bottle
no deposit no return

moving to keep warm
too cold to sleep

Leave of Abstinence

sometimes the loud of the hammer
drowns out the noise from sore backs

a careful graduate student by day
a drug rehab technician on weekend nights

the clock says three o'clock
time enough

a quiet drink
or more
and three
doctor sponsored pills
or more

set the red
alarm sober enough clock
two hours time
before work

fooling street wise drug addicts
part of the job

coming to the door
pulling me up for drug use

hospital stay follows (rehab)
back on the job in six weeks

To love a cat

an empty but still sticky CAT FOOD CAN
becomes a temporary toy

cats toss cotton in the air
then catch it
then wrestle it
then eat parts of it
so aloof
yet spends hours in magnum naps
on warm pillows or warm laps
makes no difference

Food on the table is food in a bowl
just high enough to jump
the turkey
too big for the cat to eat
but ready to lick anyway

Standing in the water dish
batting at shadows
licking bubbles

Get used to waking up
with a cat nose on your nose
and loud purring

when you bring a gift home for the cat
keep the box
that's what the cat will play with

One Man Journey

a sharp old fashioned razor
once used in barber shops

four different bottles of sleeping pills and tranquilizers
all four filled and saved
with doctor blessings

a loaded pistol
two bottles of grain alcohol
lemon juice for flavor

car packed with clean clothes
note left for wife
map to Georgia
hotel reservation
It's just off I-75
credit card with enough money
it doesn't matter why
it never really does

at least four ways
quite enough

Silent Quiet Rain

Silent rain falls inside as well as outside the walls

nurse witicker (no caps please)
Offering meds

no meds
not anymore
time spent inside red and white candy
that is bitter when chewed
run to the white room
cough up the latest drug offering
instead

Billy Jerry comes arms closed
when you won't take it by mouth
there are other ways to go
stuck with a needle stick with a thumb

so take it
go to the water tub
turn on the tub
sound hidden by silent door
tub runneth over
strange no drain
water will be up to here

I should be grateful pension and health care all covered
contributions some one else will pay
just like the pension

Carl is all right
he understands my crazy words
and can at least think
about the right things
The exercise room is open

one bag you can hit ten thousand times
take that nurse
of course a count goes in the book

tiny nurse Phillips
can leg press two hundred pounds
yet only here

She uses strength to hide from daily spouse abuse
it is the source of her gentle self
the guests think of her as number one
she is

Nurse Walters
carry a hypodermic loaded needle
in case a fire starts

one of the guests igniting
the muscled orderlies come in
a shot to the arm

a moment of peace
for the guest
and the hosts
a hazy peace for the guest

Red Napkin

There is a lady
who owns two things
one a shopping cart filled with plastic bags
and everything she knows

The bag in the front shares space with a hotel bible
a three year old Farmers Almanac
and a book of word puzzles half completed

In the quietest place in the darkest spot
near the back by two old shoes
right size but unmatched colors

One dollar and fifty cents
in aluminum cans
Forty cents in bottle redemptions
a $2.00 lottery winning ticket
donated by a rich man

hidden at the bottom in the back
 a red napkin with green letters

best of luck
Ted and Amy
20th wedding anniversary

folded into a split sided wrinkled plastic wallet
hiding tears behind the cart
many years of tears too poor to cry out loud

Red Napkin 2

inside an envelope carefully folded
a red napkin with raised green lettering

Best of Luck
Ted and Amy
20th wedding anniversary

morning meeting announcement
hospital closing budget cuts
good news you're going to independent living
property bag in tow
Rehab money runs out
Not close to retirement Social Security not yet

Welfare denied no kids
no food stamps
no room no apartment
husband left too soon heart attack eleven years ago

homeless Annie Maye Forsight
taught Amy the ways of the street
(faking alcohol addiction)
warm bed in Detox for three days per month
which dumpsters had food
sleeping under newspapers
finding shelter in furniture boxes
using plastic bags as rain coats

the route that all homeless follow

head smashed against the brass sign
crying lady
abusive spouse
stop the bus
call the cops

grabbing his wrist
stop ....Bozo

Bozo mouths off
mind you...r own business
I'll kick your ass fucker

not afraid of any man who beats
on a woman half his size

the police get there
says thank you
knows I stopped a beating

now Bozo is in cuffs
the paramedic bandages the broken head

so maybe this one gets to court
but the beating won't stop yet

Sometimes
The spouse leaves
After the first beating
Sometimes
But not often enough

Tampa Dreaming

Late at night.
When sleepy trees peak in through the window
The wind carries the sound of palm trees.

I think, of your sun colored skin.
Remembering the sand running past muscled legs
the sun flowing over your same colored hair.

A quiet kiss
a gentle squeeze
a hope of things
of the earth
hope of person

No statue could outshine you
no wind could charm you away

late night
the secret words

the difference in lovemaking at night
as opposed to in noon day Sun
is sunburn

Tampa dreams are always true
years beyond the days

Slow Clouds

Sometimes God puts God's face in the clouds
the chill of February
inhale the deep cold air
a glorious day to be bone cold
A little
cold tear in the eye

like blue skies covered with splashes of clouds

feeling numb in parts
the calm of winter trees
jagged with ice lines
sun pushes fire light
alive in ice
diamonds in the cold

somehow
the cold
looks warm

rumble and rumble
go the thick clothes
hands protected by three thumbs

close eyes
and see more lights/home

ice has the deepest warmth
The calm wind is asleep

The sound of the rails

Alone with memories
she could have waited
but our time was short by choice

The L&N Bridge
carries dull red trains
the sound of the rails
the sound of the rails
the sound of the rails

a harmonica keeps time to the train wheels
its player a resident in a red box car
with the door opened

There was a family
or loose imitation of one
brothers hurting sisters

father hurting daughters
no worry
no conscience

each brother at least one felony
daughters
charm brothers and other relatives
into bed
just the family way (incest is best)

Where is the train going?

The sound of the rails
The sound of the rails
The sound of the rails

Word Salad

"OHNO doesn't mean cat
salafras keys now
cocolumo Jesus word
Asssafras sitting now
Sit Roll malafax to ZEEBRA
Jesus
Jesus
don't never eat a tin can
balols are on the bulls
4 6 7 8 9 0 8888
a k r v f h g f
hat that cat rat fat
Oh Jsus
Salad
Jezus
Jeejes
Jesus"

Don't know
what the old man is saying
but he's talking to the right person

Your candle
has light past present and future
sometimes blurred
sometimes hazy
sometimes God

Ward

They're afraid that Mitchell
will be released and held accountable
every now and then he would disappear and go downtown
once we saw him on TV downtown dancing

Susan has a baby smothering past
Shirley pushed her mother down a flight of stairs

Peg's main problem is she is blind
and addicted to twenty years of pharmaceuticals

Sidney uses fuck and kill you in almost every sentence
she is a newcomer
only been here seven years

average IQ 52 some barely verbal

Duke once circled the day room
dragging two orderlies behind him
while he smashed glass windows
with his other fist.

An intern candidate quietly whispers to me
don't leave me alone with the patients

some brain scars left from lobotomies
much confusion caused by therapeutic brain shocks
dull physical activity
safe dosage of modern pills

a long working life with no retirement

Ward 2

Staff mad that the Recreation Therapist
wants to hold a party
for both wards
on FRIDAY at night

well usually BINGO and movies
are done in the afternoon
why have the party at night?

Party AT night has a La Masonite Cake
and real soft drinks
the diet specialist will take care of that

patients
doing dancing
voice impersonations
little political speeches
some about nurses

One routine convenes
that does a skit
the crux of it is that
if you are good
say your prayers
and treat people right
when you die
you'll go to Kentucky

they laugh they cry they plead they bargain they play they flirt they
love they hurt they miss they wish and they are forgotten

Forties

no state Hawaii
no state Alaska
no Cincinnati TV

no zip codes to carry mail
no area codes to speed up phone calls
radios played stories, plays, and news

World War II was barely over
Jet planes were just invented

Hateful No Blacks   No Negroes signs
Nasty Whites Only signs
Green River Regulations
God is still mad about those
Separate But Unequal Schools

Six computers in the whole world
Car companies were making cars instead of tanks
Korea was beginning to make World War Again

Women wore hats in church and most other times
Some men wore hats all the time

A million veterans went to school
Gandhi was assassinated
Israel became a country
The coins were silver
The first Boomers were born

Bad Manners

The sign says will work for food

Dirty hands bring a dirty rag and a bottle of vinegar
in an offer to clean my windshield
if I give a dollar
quick enough
he will go away

will work for food
likely story
he knows you don't have work for him to do
he knows you have a few dollars

I guess it all doesn't go for booze
would be a better sign
but then
sleeping in a cold deserted house
hunting for cans in the weeds
earns a bottle of red wine
or bottle of cold medicine

buddie I can see you're handicapped too
you're sure to help another vet

well I do help a handicapped vet
everyday I work
money goes to the downed man anyway
the really needy are among bad manners

just in case
just in case

Balloons Balloons

he was a silent ragged but clean man
who blew up balloons to show kids?

sometimes he would make a balloon
have mouths and ears
or tails
balloons
he only gave away balloons when the
parent was there
and the parent agreed

sometimes change or even a bill would be given
to the balloon man
he lived in an outside room that was part of a garage

the old lady only charged him $18.00 a week
it was a small room with a shower Jon and hot plate
and she liked having someone nearby at nights

balloon man lived on a small disability pension
the doctors said the brain damage
was not life threatening
but talking would be difficult
work impossible

he learned to speak
with blue and red and yellow balloons
pull them from a pocket
and shape them for a treat without words

a silent
"you are special"
to each and every kid

Balloons Balloons 2

he often listened to the radio
hearing words he could never say

had a daughter out in Arkansas
she visited last year
sent him a card every Christmas
he kept each one

every Monday he went to the library
to read the Sunday paper

sometimes he would look through the magazines
especially those with pictures
one thing he missed in life was
a marriage
and kids

So each day
down by the park
a small crowd sometimes only two
would gather waiting patiently
for the magic balloons of the balloon man

fingers turning plastic
into a laughing monkey
or a happy cow
making smiles on young faces
each balloon a story
and a smile

Sleepy Streets

walking through the sleepy streets
the soft shoes make a gentle swish on the bricks
keep walking
don't stop don't wait

sirens wake up the night
sirens begin
about the same time the bars close

the bridge over the river smells tired
used to be
I didn't have to run across bridges
hoping to outrun
the urge to jump

here and there
another man or woman
ignores me
as I wish

the secret is
there is no secret
sometimes the loss seems real

lost lovers
lost jobs
lost money
lost home
lost hope
long walks

but sister

Up most of the night
reading world book "m"
light given to me by dad

did my homework during recess
I know my handwriting is messy
I practiced for an hour on Sunday
I missed Superman

I know you're mad because I beat
Terri on the Math tests
after all she's two grades older
and her father is a doctor

I can't sleep some nights
some days I don't get hungry
I'll do the children's donation books right after recess
I'm finishing the Tom Swift book at recess

I know we're too poor
for me to go to college
but that's not till after high school anyway
Is my Dad really going to hell?
just because he's not Catholic

I can do better give me a chance

I don't want Jesus up on the cross longer
because of me

Most Excellent Dog

legs in the air

on his back

adopted a kitten
did motherly kitten duties as well

eating people food
always ready for more
eats like it is a contest

comes when called
sometimes
knows where the bed is
all the time

Chases ducks on the lake
and into the water
loves watermelon, corn on the cob and grapes
but don't call him vegetarian

call him Curly

He does not fetch
never wanted the ball anyway

Tongue out
sideways panting
his way of saying Hi, how are you?

Loves to take baths
especially the shaking off part

Most excellent dog
a most excellent friend

Awake

Time has not counted for weeks

the worst comes from nothing
nothing sleep
nothing clear thoughts
nothing energy

night time
is just more time to be awake

time is friend and foe
inside head stopped days ago

awake dreams reality numb dreams reality
pretty much the same thing

ragged thoughts hide joy
time stops but never ends

dreaming comes without sleep
split between awake self and asleep self
dreams are invisible and still seen
dreams are in color
but mostly the wrong ones

somebody said take aspirin and you'll sleep
but how many bottles?/?/?

Just a Minute Dear

I have learned to stand alone
sometimes against real odds
I have learned to need nothing (it seemed)

I stood strong (it seemed)

somehow you changed all that
knowing that your laugh
can make the hard things
pass

partner

friend

lover

spouse

seeing you at noon day
and midnight dark
brings a peace

your presence is my strength
your words are my wisdom
your voice is my light
(it seems)

take this job and love it

Sometimes the water comes in
and the broken glass
forms a new word

the reader can see the new words
and their unhidden meanings
the poet's job is simple
write with/from the soul

Some poets make money especially
with rhyming words in songs
and again
the words matter

long is the love affair
between poets and readers

a poet does not just want to "poet"
a poet has to want words to become gifts
a poet captures people places things
and shares them

shared light brightens far more than one

broken glass tracks tears and laughter and thoughts

sometimes every thing written Seems 1ike Crap
some of it is
some times only the reader can tell the difference

Bus Rider

she was always seated first seat behind the driver
all of her questions and statements were for him to hear
that used to be Steinbergs
they wouldn't give me a job

she tugs her sweater causing her ample breasts to form a V
a quiet crooked smile and eye blink
showed she used to feel sexy long ago

she looks around to catch stares
and give a dismissal look
a shrug of shoulders
and joyless smile all teeth

there wasn't a real job there anyway
Steinbergs is probably Jewish isn't it
I could never work for a Jew

the next street
had an Irish saloon
says she
the Irish bars always smell bad

the next block had a sign for fortune telling
and a huge eye
gypsies don't stay long around here

the next block was her stop
but she often stayed on to make a few rounds
the patient driver tolerates
and watches his driving
never answers her question
and she goes on next question

Bus Rider 2

She goes to Mass each Sunday
every Christmas got a three week job wrapping presents
at Kohl's Department Store
it was her only job
she had wrapped presents since High School
one of the few things she learned while in school

her reading of the newspaper was slow
mostly she read about the pictures
she listened to WBNG the jazz station

she talked to the clerk at the vegetable store
but she saved complaints for others
her look was that of anger
her voice was uneven and bitter

should anyone love her
she would get even with bitter words
would stop any approval
she rides the bus
she rides and rides and rides

the bus driver never kicked her off the bus
her bus accepted the monthly pass
so the bus was her job
Forty Eight Weeks per Year

riding route no 8 usually
sometimes an excursion
on another route
but always back to number 8
alone

Rest Stop in St Augustine, Florida

See America................greyhound 20 day bus pass
a three hour layover

a hidden place by the rush of the sea
a bottle of fruity wine
and beef jerky for dinner

the city lights are filtered by palm trees
there is a quiet song in my head

somehow your image has glowing edges
it took me thirty years
to meet you
something joyful

before I was a bastard
in action not hereditary
you would have to be crazy to hook up

midnight, the distant sparkle of starlight
would it be if you were here?
face bright with sparkly eyes

and I can't
get it out of my head
almost tears of joy

A freighter echoes a greeting
the fog rolls in

your smile I see with closed eyes
soon I will never have to go away

Mail Box

I got approved to be a million dollar winner
bulk mail permit 67543

My wife got a preapproved cemetery plot
now she can not be afraid to die

The next envelope contains a form
that declares I have been declared a member
according to laws set down by congress

another letter declares me to be
an approved member
just for getting a subscription

the next letter guarantees a month of life insurance
for only $1.00
I have to know what month I'm going to die in I guess

Another letter and another and another
comes with a nickel taped to it
all I need is 200,000 more like it

another guarantees me to be officially approved
it doesn't say on the outside what for
so I'll never know

In come for free
calendars, notebooks, name tags, note pads, name and address
labels, Christmas gift wrap, pens, candles, coins, foreign coins,
stickers, Christmas cards, ID cards, pencils, saints' pictures,
calendars, Sympathy cards, Inspirational Books, Flower seeds,
stamps, pictures, posters and Holy Rosaries

Ark the herald angels sing

What if Noah
had misunderstood God
and took extra people on the Ark

And God said to Noah
you have defied me
and I shall make leaks in the Ark

by turning the gopher wood into balsa wood
and the creosote into tissue paper

the Ark did fall apart
and it was on the twelfth day
not the fortieth the Bible says
and that is the end of this Genesis

but then could there be other genesis books?
after all the bible says
all the other folks were killed???

did not a bird come back to the Ark?
carrying a branch of peace and hope?
could it mean there were other dry spots?
besides the Ark???

did everyone get wet?
even in the desert???
how could forty days and nights flood the world?
the monsoon lasts longer

Vegetable Stew Secret Recipe

so God did not like the vegetable stew
that Cain gave him
but God liked Able

Cain killed Able
setting a precedent for vegetarians to follow

and just after God wanted to know
how Adam and Eve knew they were naked

hey dude it's pretty easy to tell
the snake told us
if we had clothes we'd be like the gods
God answered

"out of the pool"
"know death sickness work war childbirth worry"
"and the snake will crawl from now on"

well he never had legs anyway

so Adam and Eve went to work
has God regretted creating free will ever since?

Night Moods Loosely

the dark crescendo (in a loud voice) blots out
the safety of daylight
invisible rodents scamper in the blackness

the shadows almost need names
too brief to get to know too

to as in the direction
two as in how many
too to the additional

To Two Too. All three in a sentence
made up at night instead of sleep

in the direction of the two things in addition to the others
north east west and south
n.e.w.s.
News from all directions

how come the news people didn't think of that?
foolish sayings
in light of better wits

reading is possible
the early hours of not sleeping
then words begin to echo across the page
logic begins to stumble
the car won't go up the hill

Blue Wind

There is a blue wind
that pulls and pushes the face

it begins in a lonely bedroom by the ocean
and continues
to just outside of a crying man's window

each stop gives the wind a little more speed
and a little more bluer

by a lady
walking
a husband gone

past a lonely dog
rejected by a crowded family

past a new kitten
scrounging for a meal

it is a lonely wind
barely blue
to bitter
teeth bracing cold

the veteran sleepless ones
can see the blue wind just before dawn

Light Violet Sky

the new smell of dry leaves
and old grass
an unstopping blue sky
backpack and duffel bag
all I own

This place is a smiling building
old building but still useful
quite enough for the freshwomen and freshmen

long lines for registration
long lines for the hamburger shop
full computer room

current movies in the school theater
long lines in the bookstore
long lines for registration

Coffee House on Friday Night
student health insurance
bowling alley

classes
yes, go to classes at least once a week

Cafeteria
thousands of opinions
library with six Million books
writing for the student newspaper

University

naked air hammer

left arm cannot move
right hand can only move fingers
chest strap slows breathing
legs down fast in leather straps

timer on the wall
can only be strapped down two hours
staff orderly reading by the door
regs say staff must observe at all times

they call it time out
maybe they think it's grade school

it's said that isometric exercise can give you super strength
maybe I'll get back in restraints tomorrow

meds will change now

I'll probably lose canteen privileges
maybe Dr Ali will help me out

the only place you can hit somebody and not go to jail
well restraints are like jail
but restraints don't last as long as jail

some people die here
some take more pills
some get electro shock treatments
some go into restraints

Prayer of an Altar Boy

Oh God
Help me to quit being bad.
I want father S\Samuelson
to not think about me as bad.

father
He could quit hurting me
He says it would be a sin for me
to talk about it
that the devil wanted me to talk about it

I don't want to sin
but sometimes even a priest can do wrong stuff
that will hurt me
I think it is wrong

I just had one drink of communion wine

so far he's punished me three times
every time he punishes me he cries out like a little baby

none of the nuns would understand/care
father S. once whipped a boy with an extension cord
the nuns just watched

maybe some times
I would take the whipping
instead of the father S's special punishment
sometimes

Middle Mania Memories

make me laugh so I can cry
surely they are the same thing

So ask me
what picture is on page 356 in the 1946 World Book Encyclopedia?
how many I beam bridges does Ky have?
what year was radio invented?
what city has three of the five tallest TV Towers?
what do bicycles and airplanes have in common?
what three US presidents have Cincinnati Metro connections?
Abraham Lincoln did not even come second in his votes
from KY his birth state

pacing short circle small room
bed is by the sink
radio is the TV
bath is shower only
wall covered with poems

walking three miles in the city after the bars close
name and street name and town and county name all the same
no phone
closest phone is outside
hard to make loving phone calls in freezing weather

make me laugh so I can cry
surely they are the same thing
middle mania memories not for me?

Active pace pace active
pace by pace by pace
by circles

Doctors Nurses and Saturday Night

Sandy Watson
she jumped from three stories up
broke both legs
and her kidneys

George drove his car into a wall
no seat belt
but the man
had lost his job, and car and home
the air bag saved him anyway

John McWilson
he took two bottles of sleeping pills
Dead On Arrival
he made death happen

Mr Rose has a mangled arm
with 42 stitches
holds up his wrist
points to his watch and says
still running

John Bayes
wants to know if his trunk was still locked
after he was rear ended by a truck
Actually the trunk was now part of the back seat
because of the trunks huge size and speed

all in the ER

Joy Stuff

A radio that brings in Texas and New York
real black raspberry ice cream
a cat that sleeps on your nap

the laugh of a little boy
who's been given a new red car

two people promising love for keeps
while two groups watch them

Halloween masks
ex-President who builds houses for the poor

finishing a really good book
3D on TV
poems in a new voice

a dog that sleeps by the fireplace
birds that eat on a hanging bird feeder
snow ice and blue sky

Harmonica Music
new hot bread with butter
a baby "talking"

a joyful time
goes with these

Mr Woodruffs Bag

the other patients liked to tease Mr Woodruff
who always carried a black leather bag in it was a broken
stethoscope, a red alarm clock an old torn Pete Rose baseball
card, all the candy bar wrappers he had eaten that year a picture of
his dead mother, a note from his father 22 years old, and other
things

sometimes the other patients would steal the bag and hide it
Mr. Woodruff would yell and scream that he was looking for his bag
the patients would hide it in the tub room
Woodruff every time would search everywhere
the day room, the kitchen, the outside shed even other patients'
wardrobes if he could find them open
some staff would not tell him where the bag was hidden.

walking at high speed
arms forming a bag image
I want my bag, I want my bag I want my bag
he would ask staff if they saw his bag
staff persons knew the probable location
some would not tell him where to look

Mr Ron would always tell him where he had to look
and Woodruff found it.
Now counting the candy bar wrappers should be 175
now the pictures all six of them three crayon stubs, and all the rest.
Mr Woodruff would carry his bag and sometimes

would tell everybody what was in it
and years pass for Mr woodruff

Bowl of Soup

a rest from the cold street
and crowded noise
pray and stay
should be if you pray you get to stay
captive no liquor out by 8 AM to look for work

torn sweat shirt audience
mocking sermon
you know you're going to hell if you live
but don't worry
a man two thousand years ago did your time

testify not like to a quiet man in a box
but
upfront where they can hear and see
and pray for you

this pamphlet knows how to cure drinking
it was written by brother Rayburn
with the spirit of the holy ghost

if Jesus were here today
would he have to pray/beg for a bowl of soup?

Just a bowl of soup?

Freud Musings What the heck is a musing?

Freud says
sucking on a cigarette
represents sexual tension

but because a cigar is bigger
and a man sucks it
does that mean?

bigger because it's a cigar

anyone who smokes cigars
usually tells other people
don't start smoking
it's too hard to stop
then goes back to the bigger cigar

Freud said
women have no part
and that's another Freud musing
so
women are condemned
to a life of envy

but can't a woman smoke a cigar

About the poems

Many of these poems are grounded in reality. In addition to having been a Counselor, Social Worker and Mental Health Technician the writer is a Lifelong Bipolar. Successfully he has enjoyed over thirty years of relative sanity thanks to hardworking nurses and psychiatrists and of course some remarkable advances in Bipolar medicines. That is the source of some of the happy and playful poems

The poems about depression, insomnia, mania, mixed episodes, suicide, homelessness and drug abuse are all based in real life experiences. The poems on schizophrenia, dual diagnosed mental illness, spouse abuse, child molestation, religion abuse, and Drug Addiction are based on observation and/or clinical experience. So the poems are real. These are real people with real lives. In some cases several people or incidents were combined. Anonymous is how the subjects will remain. No one is tied to a real name or place. All the real parts have been sufficiently fictionalized to guarantee anonymity. Some of the poems relay the message: "you can be as bad as this and still survive and get well." The soft poems say: "You can get well and enjoy life.

Getting Help

Suicide

. Often someone will begin to contemplate suicide. This is serious. There is no such thing as a harmless wish for death.

If you are thinking about suicide it is time to get help.

Some very good and successful people have thought of or attempted suicide. The vast majority of people who get help and avoid death are glad they did. To Get Help do the following.

-Get a paper and pencil handy

-Call 1 800 273 8255

Or Call 211 Or call 911.

-Tell them that you are thinking about suicide or that you want to die

-They deal with this all the time. Everything you say is confidential and most likely the listener has dealt with similar situations before.

-Answer their questions. Be blunt and open up. It will get easier the more you talk about it.

-They will help you figure out what to do.

-Write down the steps to take.

-Follow the steps.

-If you chicken out or forget something go back and call again. They are used to people having trouble putting a plan into action.

-Accept that you are a victim. You have done nothing wrong. Get help. Live

Depression

-You are not sleeping more than a couple of hours. Or you sleep all day and night.

-You have little interest in food. Or you find yourself eating non stop.

-You are angry a lot

-You wish you did not exist.

-You think of yourself as not mattering or not being important.

-You lack energy for almost no reason.

You could be Clinically depressed.

Do the following:

-Jot down your notes of what you are going through.

-Call 211

-Tell them you think you are depressed.

-Answer the Questions they will give you.

-Tell them about your feelings, your sleep, your eating, your sense of self worth.

-Your symptoms are familiar with them. What you say is a trusted confidence.

-What they will do is help you decide what local Doctor, Hospiital. Agency, Organization can help in your area.

-They may give you other things to try.

-Write down the information.

-Begin to follow the instuctions right away.

Depression hits everywhere. Any Age, Any Occupation. If you are depressed you are a victim. You deserve help. Accept that you can be helped and things will begin to get better. Depression is treated with medicine and counseling. Both are needed. Depression works hand in hand with suicide. Often someone who is clinically depressed will begin to contemplate suicide. This is serious. There is no such thing as a harmless wish for dearh.

Mania

Mania can involve any or many of these.

-You have a hard time sitting down

-You find yourself to be impatient of many things and anyone.

-You are hiding anger a lot

-You are not sleeping your regular hours

-You are not hungry

-You are feeling superior in many things

-you feel like you can do anything

-You are spending a lot of money

-You have an unusual urge to gamble

-You have Racing unresting thoughts.

You may be having a manic episode

Do this

-Write down the unusual items you are experiencing.

-Make a list of your current daily activities.

-Dial 211

-Tell them you may be having a manic episode.

-Answer their questions.

-Write down their recommendations.

-Follow them

-Get a friend to monitor you

Bipolar Disorder

-You may be having some of the same experiences as those with a manic or depressed episode. Mania is paired with Depression to indicate a paired relationship. However some disorders may be mixed or rapid in switching.

-It is not mandatory that you experience both symptoms. If you have a Depressed Mood or Manic episode you need help.

-Write down a few symptoms

-Call 211. Tell them what you are experiencing. Answer questions. Write down steps.

-Follow the steps.

-Get a friend to help monitor your symptoms.

-Manic Depressive, Bipolar Disordered patients are often of high IQ and creative. Get help. You need it. In this disorder a little help goes a long way. People who have been involved in severe psychosis can go on to lead fulfilling lives. Don't give up.

Destructive Sleep Disorder

This form of Clinical Depression is characterized by periods of severe sleep deprivation. Sleep deprivation has been used in torture practices to rob people of their basic sanity. If you are getting only a couple of hours or less for a number of days you will begin to have painful experiences.

-Time becomes harder to appreciate.

-Long hours of deprivation can lead to distorted perceptions of space, time, sound, vision and self-awareness.

-Soon suicide begins to feel like an option.

-Some victims go for a month or longer with no more than one or two or fewer hours of sleep.

-The longer sleep is deprived the more likely sensations become distorted. In some cases the victim may intentionally or "accidently" do harm to themselves.

-It should be determined that the cause of the sleep deprivation is basically depression. But getting sleep is the first step. Nowadays there are sleep inducing medications that cause sleep but have little danger of abuse.

-Write down your sleep patterns and the way you are seeing things.

-Call 211

-Tell them you are having severe sleep disorders.

-Write down their recommendations

-Follow them.

-Getting sleep is the first step. Further counseling is needed.

411

-The phone company has a number that allows you to look up information on Psychiatrists, Emergency Rooms, Hospitals, Counseling Services, Family Doctors, Support Groups, and

Family Doctor or Nurse

Your first step in getting help may be your family doctor or nurse. Be direct and honest on what is happening with you. Tell them about sleep, eating, activity, thoughts, thoughts of suicide, how you are feeling, how you are seeing things. It is a time to be as honest as possible. The doctor or nurse may prescribe medicine and recommend another resource. Be sure you know how to get to the help usually the office staff will help you understand the resources and help you make arrangements. Don't be afraid to ask them to arrange an appointment. Use the resources of your usual health care person. YOU are the reason all the nurses, doctors, technical staff, hospitals exist. YOU deserve to be helped.

Support Groups

There are support groups for many problems including alcohol problems, obesity, bipolar disorders, depression, impaired cognition, suicide wishes...... 211 and local hospitals usually are aware of support groups in the area. Some groups are very good and some are very bad. You will have to go and see.

Notes

Buy this book $10.00

by mail
$10.00 + $2.00 postage packaging
check, money order, cash, travelers checks
Multiple copies orders (3 or more) free postpaid shipping

Title Dr, Ms, M or Mr_____   Price $10.00
                                   Postage $2.00
Name $12.00
First_____   No of copies _____
Last_____   Total Cost   _____
Address_____
Address_____

City_____ State____

Zip_____   Attention_____

Visa__ Master Charge__ Discover__ American Ex__

Account No_____
Expiration Date ____ _____
Personal 3 digit number____
Clean Table Books
1905 Alexandria
Highland Heights, KY 41076

State Sales Tax paid by Clean Table Books

Email: CTBooksAndCDs@gmail.com: www.CTBooksAndCDs.com

Emergency Contacts

Person	Phone Number
Suicide Hotline _____	1 800 273 8255
General Help _____	**211**_____
Emergency_____	911_____
Phones_____	411_____

_____

_____

_____

_____

_____

_____

_____

_____

_____

_____

_____

_____

_____

Medical Notes

Person   Note

_____   _____

_____   _____

_____   _____

_____   _____

_____   _____